SOMATIC YOGA WORKOUT

5 Minutes Low Impact Exercises To Lose Weight Fast And Treat Trauma, Pain And Relief Stress

DR. PERSIS HILLARY

TABLE OF CONTENTS

5. Neck Stretches

6. Spinal Twists

7. Child's Pose

8. Hip Circles

9. Leg Lifts

10. Arm Sweeps

11. Knee to Chest Stretch

12. Ankle Rolls

13. Side Bends

14. Cobra Pose

15. Seated Forward Bend

16. Mountain Pose

17. Knee Sways

18. Balancing Table Pose

19. Gentle Backbends

20. Butterfly Pose

21. Supine Spinal Rotation

22. Bridge Pose

23. Warrior I Pose

24. Warrior II Pose

25. Extended Triangle Pose

26. Tree Pose

27. Downward Facing Dog

28. Pigeon Pose

29. Camel Pose

30. Corpse Pose (Savasana)

31. Seated Twist

32. Happy Baby Pose

33. Standing Forward Bend

34. Half Lord of the Fishes Pose

35. Eagle Pose

INTRODUCTION

The Concept of Somatic Yoga

Somatic Yoga, emerging from the intersection of somatic education and traditional yoga, is a holistic approach that emphasizes internal physical perception and experience. The word "somatic" is derived from the Greek term "soma," meaning the living body in its wholeness. This form of yoga focuses not just on the physical postures (asanas) but on the deep, integrative experience of movement and breath.

In Somatic Yoga, the emphasis is placed on the awareness of the internal state of the body. It prioritizes gentle movements, mindfulness, and the connection between mind and body. This approach is deeply rooted in the understanding that our mental and emotional states are intrinsically linked to our physical well-being. Somatic Yoga practitioners often engage in movements that are aimed at releasing tension and restoring natural movement patterns, fostering a heightened sense of body awareness.

Benefits of Somatic Yoga

The benefits of Somatic Yoga are multifaceted, addressing both physical and mental health. One of the primary advantages is improved body awareness. Practitioners learn to notice subtle cues from their bodies, which can lead to better posture, reduced tension, and a more harmonious relationship with their physical selves.

On a physical level, Somatic Yoga can lead to increased flexibility, strength, and mobility. The gentle, mindful approach makes it particularly beneficial for those recovering from injuries or dealing with chronic pain. It helps in re-educating the muscles and the nervous system to release chronic muscle tension and improve movement efficiency.

Mentally, Somatic Yoga offers a pathway to stress reduction and emotional balance. The practice encourages mindfulness and present-moment awareness, which can reduce anxiety and promote a sense of calm. It also fosters a meditative state that can lead to deeper self-awareness and emotional release.

How to Use This Book

This book is designed to be both a guide and a companion in your journey through Somatic Yoga. Whether you are a beginner or an experienced yogi, the content is structured to cater to various levels of experience and understanding.

1. Foundational Concepts: Begin with the foundational concepts of Somatic Yoga. This section offers a deep dive into the philosophy and principles underlying this practice. Understanding these concepts is crucial for a meaningful and effective practice.

2. Practical Techniques: The book provides detailed descriptions and illustrations of specific Somatic Yoga techniques and sequences. These are designed to guide you through the movements and postures, helping you to practice safely and effectively.

3. Mind-Body Integration: Special emphasis is placed on integrating mind and body. This section includes exercises and meditations that focus on developing body awareness and mindfulness, essential components of Somatic Yoga.

4. Personalizing Your Practice: Recognizing that every individual is unique, the book offers guidance on tailoring your Somatic Yoga practice to your specific needs, goals, and physical condition.

5. Progressive Learning: The book is structured to facilitate progressive learning. You can move through the chapters sequentially or focus on areas that particularly interest you.

6. Reflective and Interactive Elements: Throughout the book, there are prompts for reflection and spaces for journaling your experiences. This interactive element is designed to deepen your understanding and personal connection to the practice.

This book aims to provide a comprehensive and enriching experience of Somatic Yoga, guiding you through a journey of physical and mental transformation.

CHAPTER 1: UNDERSTANDING SOMATICS

1. The Philosophy of Somatics

Somatics, at its core, is a field that emphasizes the importance of the body in understanding and experiencing the world. This philosophy contends that the mind and body are not separate entities but are intricately interconnected. In somatics, the body is not just a vessel for the mind but an integral part of our being that influences and is influenced by our mental and emotional states.

This approach challenges traditional Western notions that often place a higher value on the mind and intellectual pursuits, suggesting that bodily experiences are just as crucial in shaping our identity and perception of the world. Somatics encourages a holistic view of human existence, where physical sensations, movements, and bodily experiences are seen as fundamental components of life that contribute to our understanding of ourselves and our surroundings.

2. Somatics and Body Awareness

Body awareness is a key concept in somatics. It refers to the conscious perception and understanding of one's body, including its position, movement, and the interplay of its various parts. Somatic practices aim to enhance this body awareness, allowing individuals to become more attuned to their physical sensations and movements.

This heightened awareness is believed to lead to a deeper understanding of oneself. It can foster improved movement patterns, greater ease and efficiency in physical activities, and a reduction in physical discomfort and stress. By becoming more aware of the subtle cues of the body, individuals can also gain insights into their emotional and psychological states, as the body often manifests internal experiences in physical ways.

3. The Connection between Mind and Body

The mind-body connection is a pivotal aspect of somatics. This concept posits that the mind and body are dynamically linked, each constantly influencing the other. Emotional and psychological states can manifest physically, as seen in phenomena like stress-induced headaches or the physical exhaustion felt after intense emotional experiences. Conversely, physical states can impact mental and emotional wellbeing.

Somatics explores this interplay through various techniques and practices. These can include movement therapies, mindful exercises, and bodywork. The goal is to harmonize the mind and body, creating a state of balance and integrated functioning. By acknowledging and working with this connection, somatic practices aim to promote overall health and wellbeing, recognizing that mental, emotional, and physical health are deeply intertwined and interdependent.

Somatics offers a comprehensive approach to understanding human existence by valuing the body as much as the mind. It emphasizes the importance of body awareness and explores the intricate connection between the mind and body to enhance wellbeing and self-understanding.

CHAPTER 2: FOUNDATIONS OF YOGA

History and Philosophy of Yoga

Yoga, an ancient practice with its roots in India, has evolved over thousands of years. It is believed to have originated during the Vedic period, around 1500 BCE, but its development spans several major eras in Indian history. Yoga is more than just physical postures; it's a comprehensive system that encompasses physical, mental, and spiritual practices.

Key philosophical texts, such as the Yoga Sutras of Patanjali and the Bhagavad Gita, have been instrumental in shaping yoga's philosophy. The Yoga Sutras, composed around 400 CE, introduce the concept of Ashtanga, or the eight limbs of yoga, which include ethics, discipline, physical postures, breath control, sensory withdrawal, concentration, meditation, and a state of blissful union. The Bhagavad Gita, part of the Indian epic Mahabharata, discusses the importance of yoga as a path to spiritual realization and the balance between action and contemplation.

Types of Yoga and Their Benefits

Yoga has diversified into various styles, each with unique characteristics and benefits:

1. Hatha Yoga: This is the most widely practiced form in the West, known for its gentle introduction to yoga postures and breathing techniques. It improves flexibility, strength, and relaxation.

2. Ashtanga Yoga: A rigorous style characterized by a series of specific postures synchronized with breath, beneficial for building core strength and toning the body.

3. Iyengar Yoga: Focuses on precision and alignment in the execution of postures. It often uses props like belts and blocks and is excellent for those with injuries or who want to improve their posture.

4. Kundalini Yoga: Combines postures, breathing exercises, and the chanting of mantras to awaken the kundalini energy at the base of the spine. It aims to improve self-awareness and provide a spiritual experience.

5. Bikram Yoga: Consists of a specific sequence of 26 postures and two breathing exercises practiced in a room heated to about 40 degrees Celsius. It's great for detoxifying the body and improving flexibility.

6. Vinyasa Flow: Known for its fluid, movement-intensive practices. Vinyasa aligns a deliberate sequence of poses with the breath to achieve a continuous flow.

Each style of yoga offers distinct benefits, from enhancing physical strength and flexibility to promoting mental clarity and stress reduction.

Yoga as a Holistic Practice

Yoga is not just a physical exercise; it's a holistic practice that integrates the body, mind, and spirit. The holistic approach of yoga emphasizes the balance between physical health, mental clarity, and emotional well-being. This integration is achieved through the combination of postures (asanas), breathing techniques (pranayama), meditation (dhyana), and ethical living.

Regular practice of yoga can lead to increased self-awareness, mindfulness, and a sense of inner peace. It encourages a deeper understanding of the self and the environment, fostering a sense of harmony and balance. Additionally, yoga's emphasis on mindfulness and living in the present moment can have profound benefits on mental health, helping to alleviate anxiety and depression.

The foundations of yoga are deeply rooted in its rich history and philosophy, offering a diverse range of practices that cater to different needs and benefits, all while maintaining its core essence as a holistic practice that nurtures the body, mind, and spirit.

CHAPTER 3: THE SOMATIC YOGA APPROACH

Integrating Somatics and Yoga

Somatics, a field concerned with the internal physical perceptions and experiences of the body, intersects intriguingly with Yoga, an ancient discipline emphasizing physical postures, breath control, and meditation. The integration of Somatics into Yoga offers a holistic approach that enhances self-awareness and internal body sensations. This fusion allows practitioners to engage more deeply with their bodies, recognizing and releasing tension and stress. By doing so, the practice of Yoga transforms from merely executing poses to a more profound journey of internal exploration and healing.

Principles of Somatic Yoga

At the core of Somatic Yoga are several key principles:

1. Body-Mind Connection: This principle emphasizes understanding the body and mind as an interconnected unit. Every movement and posture in Somatic Yoga is as much about mental and emotional awareness as it is about physical alignment.

2. Self-regulation and Healing: Somatic Yoga operates on the belief that the body possesses innate abilities for self-healing and regulation. Practices focus on activating these self-healing processes, primarily through mindful movements and awareness.

3. Gentleness and Ease: Unlike some Yoga practices that emphasize strength and endurance, Somatic Yoga advocates for gentle movements that prioritize ease and comfort, allowing for a deeper connection with the body's subtle sensations.

4. Individualized Practice: Recognizing that each body is unique, Somatic Yoga encourages a highly individualized approach. It respects personal limits and advocates for adapting poses and practices to suit individual needs.

Mindfulness in Somatic Yoga

Mindfulness is a cornerstone of Somatic Yoga. It involves a heightened, non-judgmental awareness of the present moment, particularly focusing on bodily sensations, thoughts, and emotions. In Somatic Yoga, mindfulness is practiced through:

- Attentive Movement: Practitioners are encouraged to move with full attention, noticing the sensations, emotions, and thoughts that arise with each movement.

- Breath Awareness: Breath is used as a tool to anchor the mind in the present and to deepen the connection with the body's internal state.

- Meditative Practices: Somatic Yoga often incorporates meditative practices that foster a deep state of relaxation and inner awareness, further enhancing the mind-body connection.

CHAPTER 4: PREPARING FOR YOUR PRACTICE

Setting Up Your Space

When you're preparing a space for practice, whether it's for exercise, yoga, meditation, or any other activity, the environment plays a crucial role in your experience and effectiveness. A well-set-up space can enhance concentration, comfort, and overall enjoyment. Here are key considerations:

1. Choose the Right Location: Look for an area that is quiet, free from distractions, and has enough room for movement. Natural light and good ventilation can also be beneficial.

2. Personalize Your Space: Add elements that make the space inviting and motivational. This could include plants, inspirational posters, or calming colors.

3. Organize for Efficiency: Ensure that everything you need is easily accessible. A clutter-free and well-

organized space helps in maintaining focus and flow during practice.

Essential Equipment

The equipment you need depends largely on the type of practice you are engaging in. However, there are some general pieces of equipment that are commonly useful:

1. Quality Mats or Cushions: For activities like yoga or meditation, a good mat or cushion is fundamental for comfort and stability.

2. Appropriate Attire: Wear clothing that allows for full range of motion and is suitable for the type of practice and environment.

3. Supportive Accessories: Depending on your practice, items like resistance bands, weights, blocks, or bolsters can enhance your practice.

Safety and Injury Prevention

Safety should be your top priority to ensure a sustainable and beneficial practice. Here are key guidelines:

1. Understand Your Body's Limits: Listen to your body and understand its limits. Avoid pushing too hard and recognize the difference between good pain (like muscle stretching) and bad pain (like sharp or shooting pain).

2. Warm-Up and Cool-Down: Incorporate a proper warm-up before and a cool-down period after your practice. This helps in preparing and recovering your muscles and joints.

3. Learn Proper Techniques: Whether self-taught or under guidance, ensure that you are practicing correct techniques to avoid injuries.

4. Regular Breaks and Hydration: Take breaks as needed, especially during intense sessions, and stay hydrated to maintain your body's balance.

5. Emergency Preparedness: Keep a first-aid kit handy and be aware of basic first aid procedures relevant to your practice.

By carefully setting up your space, selecting the right equipment, and prioritizing safety and injury prevention, you can create an effective and enjoyable practice routine. This preparation not only enhances the immediate experience but also contributes to long-term consistency and success in your practice.

CHAPTER 5: EXERCISES

1. Cat-Cow Stretch

Purpose: This exercise improves spinal flexibility and relieves tension in your torso.

Steps:

1. Start on Hands and Knees: Position yourself on a yoga mat with your wrists under your shoulders and knees under your hips.

2. Cow Pose: Inhale, drop your belly towards the mat, lift your chin and chest, and gaze upwards. Allow your back to curve naturally.

3. Cat Pose: As you exhale, round your back towards the ceiling, tuck in your chin towards your chest, and draw your belly to your spine.

4. Flow Between Poses: Continue this flow for several breaths, moving between Cow Pose on the inhale and Cat Pose on the exhale.

2. Pelvic Tilts

Purpose: Pelvic tilts strengthen the lower back and abdomen.

Steps:

1. Lie on Your Back: Start by lying flat on your back with your knees bent and feet flat on the floor.

2. Engage Your Core: Inhale and as you exhale, engage your abdominal muscles, tilting your pelvis towards your navel.

3. Return to Neutral: Inhale and gently return your pelvis to a neutral position.

4. Repeat: Do this slowly for several repetitions, focusing on the movement of your pelvis.

3. Diaphragmatic Breathing

Purpose: This breathing exercise reduces stress and improves oxygen flow.

Steps:

1. Comfortable Position: Sit or lie in a comfortable position.

2. Hand Placement: Place one hand on your chest and the other on your abdomen.

3. Inhale Deeply: Inhale slowly through your nose, allowing your diaphragm to expand and your abdomen to rise.

4. Exhale Slowly: Exhale through pursed lips, feeling your abdomen fall and diaphragm contract.

5. Repeat: Continue for several minutes, focusing on the rise and fall of your abdomen.

4. Shoulder Rolls

Purpose: Shoulder rolls help relieve tension and increase shoulder mobility.

Steps:

1. Start Upright: Sit or stand with your spine straight.

2. Roll Your Shoulders: Lift your shoulders up towards your ears, roll them back, down, and then forward in a smooth, circular motion.

3. Reverse Direction: After several rolls, reverse the direction and continue.

4. Relax and Repeat: Do this for a few minutes, relaxing your shoulder muscles.

5. Neck Stretches

Purpose: These stretches can help relieve neck tension and increase flexibility.

Steps:

1. Sit Comfortably: Sit in a relaxed position with your spine straight.

2. Side Stretch: Gently tilt your head towards your right shoulder, using your right hand to apply a light stretch. Hold for a few breaths, then switch sides.

3. Forward Stretch: Lower your chin to your chest to stretch the back of your neck. Hold for several breaths.

4. Backward Stretch: Tilt your head back carefully to stretch the front of your neck. Hold briefly.

5. Rotate: Slowly turn your head to look over each shoulder.

6. Repeat: Do these stretches gently, without forcing your neck into uncomfortable positions.

Certainly! Here are step-by-step instructions for each of the yoga exercises listed, presented in an original and detailed manner.

6. Spinal Twists

Spinal Twists are excellent for increasing spinal mobility and can help relieve back tension.

1. Start Seated: Sit on the floor with your legs extended in front of you.

2. Bend Your Knee: Bend your right knee and place your right foot flat on the floor on the outside of your left knee.

3. Twist Your Torso: Turn your torso to the right. Place your left elbow on the outside of your right knee and your right hand on the floor behind you for support.

4. Hold and Breathe: Hold this pose for 20-30 seconds, breathing deeply. Feel the twist in your spine.

5. Repeat on the Other Side: Unwind and repeat the same steps on the opposite side.

7. Child's Pose

Child's Pose is a restorative posture that helps to relax the body and mind.

1. Start on Your Knees: Kneel on the floor with your big toes touching and knees hip-width apart.

2. Bow Forward: Exhale and lay your torso down between your thighs, resting your forehead on the floor.

3. Extend Your Arms: Stretch your arms forward, palms down, or let them rest alongside your body, palms up.

4. Relax in the Pose: Hold for 30 seconds to a few minutes, focusing on deep, slow breaths.

8. Hip Circles

Hip Circles are great for loosening the hips and lower back.

1. Stand Firmly: Stand with your feet wider than hip-width apart, knees slightly bent.

2. Circle Your Hips: Place your hands on your hips and move your hips in a circular motion.

3. Change Directions: Do 10-15 circles in one direction, then switch and do the same number in the opposite direction.

9. Leg Lifts

Leg Lifts strengthen the abdominal muscles and improve lower body flexibility.

1. Lie on Your Back: Lie down flat on your back with your legs extended and arms by your sides.

2. Raise Your Legs: Inhale and slowly raise your legs to a 90-degree angle, keeping them straight.

3. Lower Down Slowly: Exhale and slowly lower your legs back down without letting them touch the floor.

4. Repeat: Do 10-15 repetitions.

10. Arm Sweeps

Arm Sweeps are good for improving upper body mobility and relieving shoulder tension.

1. Stand Tall: Stand with your feet hip-width apart.

2. Sweep Arms Forward and Up: Inhale and sweep your arms forward and up overhead, palms facing each other.

3. Sweep Arms Down and Back: Exhale and sweep your arms down and back, palms facing down.

4. Repeat the Motion: Continue this sweeping motion smoothly for 15-20 repetitions.

11. Knee to Chest Stretch (Apanasana)

This exercise helps in stretching the lower back and relieving tension.

1. Start Position: Lie flat on your back on a comfortable yoga mat.

2. Movement: Bend your knees and bring them towards your chest.

3. Hand Placement: Wrap your arms around your knees, holding each elbow with the opposite hand.

4. Hold and Breathe: Gently pull your knees closer to your chest. Breathe deeply and hold the position for several breaths.

5. Release: Slowly release your arms and return your feet to the floor.

12. Ankle Rolls

Ankle rolls improve flexibility and circulation in the ankles and feet.

1. Start Position: Sit comfortably with your legs extended forward.

2. Movement: Lift one foot off the ground and rotate your ankle slowly in a circular motion.

3. Direction: Rotate 5-10 times in one direction, then switch to the opposite direction.

4. Repeat: Lower the foot back to the ground and repeat with the other foot.

13. Side Bends

Side bends stretch the lateral muscles of the body and improve flexibility in the torso.

1. Start Position: Stand or sit upright with your spine straight.

2. Movement: Raise your arms overhead, interlocking your fingers.

3. Bend: Exhale and gently bend your body to one side, keeping your arms straight.

4. Hold and Breathe: Hold for a few breaths, feeling the stretch along the side of your body.

5. Return and Repeat: Inhale and come back to the center. Repeat on the other side.

14. Cobra Pose (Bhujangasana)

This pose strengthens the spine and opens up the chest and shoulders.

1. Start Position: Lie on your stomach with your toes flat and forehead resting on the ground.

2. Hand Placement: Place your hands under your shoulders, elbows close to your body.

3. Lift: Inhale and slowly lift your head, chest, and abdomen while keeping your navel on the floor.

4. Hold and Breathe: Straighten your arms as much as comfortable, tilt your head back, and breathe.

5. Release: Exhale and gently lower your abdomen, chest, and head back to the floor.

15. Seated Forward Bend (Paschimottanasana)

This pose stretches the spine, shoulders, and hamstrings.

1. Start Position: Sit on the floor with your legs stretched out in front of you.

2. Inhale: Inhale and raise your arms above your head.

3. Bend Forward: Exhale and bend forward from the hip joints, chin moving toward the toes.

4. Hand Placement: Place your hands on your legs, wherever they reach without straining.

5. Hold and Breathe: Keep your back as straight as possible, hold the position for a few breaths.

6. Release: Inhale, lift your torso, and lower your arms.

Certainly! I'll provide you with thorough and unique step-by-step instructions for each of the yoga poses you've listed. These poses are suitable for practitioners of various levels and are beneficial for improving balance, flexibility, and strength.

16. Mountain Pose (Tadasana)

1. Start Standing: Stand with your feet hip-width apart, spreading your toes wide to distribute your weight evenly.

2. Align Your Body: Engage your thighs to lift your kneecaps slightly, but avoid locking your knees. Tuck your tailbone slightly, but don't round your lower back.

3. Position Arms: Let your arms hang naturally with palms facing forward. This opens up your chest and shoulders.

4. Align Head and Neck: Keep your head in line with your spine, and your chin parallel to the floor. Gaze forward.

5. Breathe and Hold: Take deep, even breaths. Feel your body grounded and stable, like a mountain. Hold for 30 seconds to a minute.

17. Knee Sways

1. Start Lying Down: Lie on your back with your knees bent and feet flat on the floor, hip-width apart.

2. Sway Gently: Gently sway your knees from side to side, maintaining a rhythm that feels comfortable.

3. Coordinate with Breath: Inhale as your knees go to one side, and exhale as you bring them back to the center. Repeat on the other side.

4. Engage Your Core: Keep your core engaged and shoulders pressed to the floor for stability.

5. Duration: Continue for 1-2 minutes, gradually slowing down the movement.

18. Balancing Table Pose

1. Start on Fours: Begin on your hands and knees. Ensure your wrists are under your shoulders and your knees under your hips.

2. Extend Arm and Leg: Extend your right arm forward and your left leg back, keeping them parallel to the floor.

3. Focus on Balance: Engage your core for balance. Keep your head and neck in a neutral position, gazing down at the floor.

4. Hold and Switch: Hold the pose for a few breaths, then gently lower your hand and knee to the starting position. Repeat on the opposite side.

5. Duration: Do 5-10 repetitions on each side.

19. Gentle Backbends

1. Start Standing or Kneeling: You can perform a gentle backbend either standing or kneeling.

2. Hands on Hips: Place your hands on your lower back or hips for support.

3. Lean Back Gently: Inhale and gently arch your back, pushing your hips forward. Keep the movement smooth and controlled.

4. Neck Position: Keep your neck neutral or slightly extended, but don't strain it.

5. Hold and Return: Hold the backbend for a few breaths, then slowly return to the starting position. Repeat 2-3 times.

20. Butterfly Pose (Baddha Konasana)

1. Sit Down: Sit with your legs straight out in front of you.

2. Bend Knees: Bend your knees and bring the soles of your feet together, pulling them as close to your body as comfortable.

3. Open Hips: Gently press your knees down with your elbows or hands, feeling a stretch in your inner thighs.

4. Straight Back: Keep your spine straight and long. You can sit on a cushion or folded blanket to help maintain posture.

5. Breathe and Hold: Breathe deeply and hold the pose for 1-3 minutes, focusing on the stretch and relaxation.

Of course, I can provide you with unique step-by-step instructions for each of these yoga poses without plagiarizing. Let's get started:

21. Supine Spinal Rotation:

Step 1: Begin by lying flat on your back on a comfortable mat or surface.

Step 2: Extend your arms out to the sides, forming a "T" shape with your body.

Step 3: Bend your knees and bring them towards your chest, keeping your feet flat on the ground.

Step 4: Slowly lower your knees to the right side while keeping your shoulders grounded. Your knees and hips should be stacked.

Step 5: Gently turn your head to the left, looking in the opposite direction of your knees.

Step 6: Hold this position for 20-30 seconds, focusing on deep and relaxed breathing.

Step 7: Return your knees to the center and repeat the rotation on the left side.

22. Bridge Pose:

Step 1: Lie on your back with your knees bent and feet flat on the ground, hip-width apart.

Step 2: Place your arms alongside your body, with palms facing down.

Step 3: Inhale and press your feet into the ground, lifting your hips and lower back off the mat.

Step 4: Keep your thighs parallel to each other, and your knees directly above your heels.

Step 5: Engage your glutes and core muscles as you continue to lift your hips higher.

Step 6: Hold the pose for 20-30 seconds, breathing deeply.

Step 7: Exhale as you gently lower your hips back down to the mat.

23. Warrior I Pose:

Step 1: Start in a standing position at the top of your mat, with your feet hip-width apart.

Step 2: Step your left foot back, keeping it at a 45-degree angle, and bend your right knee to a 90-degree angle.

Step 3: Square your hips forward toward the front of the mat.

Step 4: Inhale as you raise your arms overhead, bringing your palms together.

Step 5: Keep your chest open and shoulders relaxed, gazing forward or slightly upward.

Step 6: Hold the pose for 20-30 seconds, breathing deeply.

Step 7: Exhale and lower your arms and step your left foot back to the starting position.

24. Warrior II Pose:

Step 1: Begin in a standing position at the top of your mat, with your feet hip-width apart.

Step 2: Step your left foot back, keeping it at a 90-degree angle, and bend your right knee to a 90-degree angle.

Step 3: Extend your arms out to the sides, parallel to the ground, with palms facing down.

Step 4: Keep your gaze fixed over your right fingertips.

Step 5: Engage your core and maintain a strong stance.

Step 6: Hold the pose for 20-30 seconds, breathing deeply.

Step 7: Exhale and return to the starting position, then switch sides.

25. Extended Triangle Pose:

Step 1: Start in a standing position with your feet wide apart, toes pointing forward.

Step 2: Turn your right foot out 90 degrees and your left foot slightly inwards.

Step 3: Inhale as you raise your arms to shoulder height, parallel to the ground.

Step 4: Exhale and reach your right hand towards your right shin or ankle, extending your left arm upwards.

Step 5: Keep your chest open, and gaze up at your left hand.

Step 6: Hold the pose for 20-30 seconds, breathing deeply.

Step 7: Inhale as you return to a standing position and repeat on the opposite side.

Sure, I can provide unique step-by-step instructions for each of these yoga poses:

26. Tree Pose (Vrikshasana):

Tree Pose is a balancing yoga posture that strengthens your legs and improves focus and concentration.

1. Begin by standing in Tadasana (Mountain Pose), with your feet hip-width apart and arms at your sides.

2. Shift your weight onto your right foot while keeping your left foot grounded.

3. Slowly lift your left foot and place the sole of your left foot against your right inner thigh, with your toes pointing downward. If you can't reach your inner thigh, you can place your foot on your calf instead.

4. Press your hands together at your chest in a prayer position or extend your arms upward.

5. Find a focal point to gaze at, which will help you maintain balance.

6. Engage your core muscles and relax your shoulders. Keep your spine straight.

7. Take a few deep breaths, and with each exhale, root down through your standing foot.

8. Hold the pose for 30 seconds to 1 minute, or as long as you can maintain balance.

9. Slowly lower your left foot back to the ground.

10. Repeat on the other side, shifting your weight to your left foot and placing your right foot against your inner thigh.

27. Downward Facing Dog (Adho Mukha Svanasana):

Downward Facing Dog is a fundamental yoga pose that stretches and strengthens the entire body.

1. Start on your hands and knees in a tabletop position, with your wrists directly under your shoulders and knees under your hips.

2. Spread your fingers wide apart and press firmly into your palms.

3. Tuck your toes under and lift your hips toward the ceiling, straightening your legs.

4. Create an inverted "V" shape with your body, keeping your back straight and lengthening your spine.

5. Press your heels toward the floor, but it's okay if they don't touch.

6. Engage your core muscles to support your lower back and keep your neck relaxed.

7. Hold the pose for 30 seconds to 1 minute, breathing deeply and evenly.

8. To release, bend your knees and return to the tabletop position.

28. Pigeon Pose (Eka Pada Rajakapotasana):

Pigeon Pose is a hip-opening yoga pose that helps relieve tension and tightness in the hips and lower back.

1. Begin in a tabletop position with your hands under your shoulders and knees under your hips.

2. Bring your right knee forward and place it behind your right wrist, angling your right shin diagonally across your mat.

3. Slide your left leg back and straighten it behind you, keeping your toes pointed.

4. Square your hips as much as possible, with your right hip facing down toward the mat.

5. Inhale to lengthen your spine, and as you exhale, walk your hands forward and lower your torso toward the mat.

6. You can rest your forearms on the ground or extend your arms in front of you.

7. Hold the pose for 30 seconds to 1 minute, breathing deeply and focusing on releasing tension in your hips.

8. Slowly come out of the pose by walking your hands back, tucking your left toes, and lifting your hips.

9. Repeat on the other side.

29. Camel Pose (Ustrasana):

Camel Pose is a heart-opening yoga pose that stretches the front of the body and improves posture.

1. Kneel on your mat with your knees hip-width apart.

2. Tuck your toes under, pressing the tops of your feet into the mat.

3. Place your hands on your lower back, fingers pointing downward, with your thumbs on your sacrum for support.

4. Inhale, engage your core, and gently arch your back, lifting your chest toward the ceiling.

5. Start to lean back, keeping your hips aligned over your knees.

6. If comfortable, reach one hand at a time toward your heels, resting them there.

7. Keep your neck relaxed and gaze at the ceiling or behind you.

8. Hold the pose for 20-30 seconds, breathing deeply.

9. To come out of the pose, bring your hands back to your lower back, and slowly lift your torso to an upright position.

10. Sit back on your heels and take a few breaths before moving on.

30. Corpse Pose (Savasana):

Corpse Pose is a relaxation and meditation pose that helps calm the mind and rejuvenate the body.

1. Lie flat on your back on your mat with your legs extended and arms at your sides.

2. Allow your feet to fall open naturally, and your arms to rest slightly away from your body with your palms facing up.

3. Close your eyes and take a few deep breaths to relax your body.

4. Focus on each part of your body, starting from your toes and moving up to your head, consciously relaxing and releasing any tension.

5. Let go of any thoughts or distractions, allowing your mind to become still.

6. Remain in Savasana for at least 5-10 minutes, or as long as you like, continuing to breathe deeply and letting go of any mental chatter.

7. When you're ready to come out of the pose, gently wiggle your fingers and toes, then roll onto your side before slowly sitting up.

31. Seated Twist:

  - Sit on the floor with your legs extended.

  - Bend your right knee and place your right foot on the outside of your left thigh.

  - Inhale and lengthen your spine.

- Exhale as you twist your torso to the right, bringing your left elbow to the outside of your right knee.

- Place your right hand on the floor behind you for support.

- Hold the twist for several deep breaths, feeling the gentle stretch in your spine and abdomen.

- Inhale to release the twist and switch sides, repeating the process on the opposite side.

32. Happy Baby Pose:

- Lie on your back with your knees bent and your feet flat on the floor.

- Exhale and bring your knees towards your chest.

- Grab the outsides of your feet with your hands, keeping your knees bent and your feet flexed.

- Gently pull your knees down towards the floor, opening your hips.

- Keep your back and shoulders on the ground as you relax into the stretch.

- Take deep breaths and enjoy the sensation of opening your hips and lower back.

33. Standing Forward Bend:

- Stand with your feet hip-width apart and your arms at your sides.

- Inhale deeply, lengthening your spine.

- Exhale and hinge at your hips, bending forward from your waist.

- Keep your back straight as you fold forward, reaching for your toes or the floor.

- If you can't touch the floor, bend your knees slightly.

- Relax your neck and let your head hang.

- Breathe deeply as you feel the stretch in your hamstrings and lower back.

- Inhale and slowly rise back up to a standing position.

34. Half Lord of the Fishes Pose:

- Sit with your legs extended in front of you.

- Bend your right knee and place your right foot on the floor outside your left thigh.

- Inhale and lengthen your spine.

- Exhale and twist your torso to the right, placing your left elbow on the outside of your right knee.

- Keep your right hand behind you for support.

- Gently twist your upper body, looking over your right shoulder.

- Breathe deeply and hold the pose, feeling the stretch in your spine and hips.

- Inhale to release the twist and switch sides.

35. Eagle Pose:

- Stand with your feet hip-width apart.

- Bend your knees slightly and shift your weight onto your right foot.

- Lift your left leg and cross it over your right thigh.

- Wrap your left foot around your right calf if possible.

- Extend your arms in front of you and cross your left arm over your right.

- Bend your elbows and bring your palms together, if possible.

- Balance on your right leg and sink down slightly into the pose.

- Breathe deeply and hold for a few breaths.

- Unwrap your limbs and repeat on the opposite side.

36. Chair Pose:

- Stand with your feet together and your arms at your sides.

- Inhale deeply.

- Exhale and bend your knees, lowering your hips as if you were sitting in an imaginary chair.

- Keep your weight in your heels and your knees over your ankles.

- Raise your arms overhead, parallel to each other or with your palms facing each other.

- Engage your core and keep your spine straight.

- Breathe deeply as you hold the pose, feeling the burn in your thighs.

- Inhale to rise back up to a standing position.

37. Sun Salutations:

Sun Salutations, also known as Surya Namaskar, are a great way to energize your body and mind. Follow these steps:

1. Stand tall at the front of your mat with your feet together and palms pressed together at your heart center, taking a moment to center yourself.

2. Inhale deeply as you raise your arms overhead, arching your back slightly, and look up at your hands.

3. Exhale as you fold forward at the hips, bringing your hands down to the mat beside your feet. If needed, you can bend your knees slightly.

4. Inhale and step your right foot back into a lunge position, keeping your left knee directly above your left ankle.

5. Exhale as you step your left foot back into a plank position, engaging your core and keeping your body in a straight line.

6. Lower your knees, chest, and chin to the mat while keeping your hips lifted. Inhale as you glide forward into Cobra Pose, arching your back and lifting your chest.

7. Exhale as you tuck your toes, lift your hips, and press back into Downward-Facing Dog.

8. Inhale and step your right foot forward into a lunge, followed by your left foot.

9. Exhale as you fold forward over your legs, keeping your back straight.

10. Inhale deeply as you rise back up, extending your arms overhead.

11. Exhale and bring your hands back to your heart center, completing one round of Sun Salutations. Repeat this sequence for a full practice.

38. Crescent Moon Pose:

Crescent Moon Pose is a wonderful stretch for the sides of your body. Follow these steps:

1. Start in a standing position with your feet hip-width apart and your arms at your sides.

2. Inhale and raise your arms overhead, interlocking your fingers and releasing your index fingers, leaving the thumbs crossed.

3. Lean to your right side, stretching your left arm up and over your head while keeping your feet firmly planted.

4. Hold the stretch for a few breaths, feeling the stretch along the left side of your body.

5. Inhale to come back to the center.

6. Exhale and lean to your left side, stretching your right arm up and over your head, again feeling the stretch along the right side of your body.

7. Inhale to return to the center.

8. Repeat the stretch to each side several times, focusing on your breath and maintaining balance.

39. Garland Pose:

Garland Pose, also known as Malasana, is excellent for stretching the hips and strengthening the lower body. Here's how to do it:

1. Begin by standing with your feet slightly wider than hip-width apart, with your toes turned slightly outward.

2. Lower your body into a squatting position, keeping your heels on the ground as much as possible.

3. Bring your palms together at your heart center, pressing your elbows against your inner knees.

4. Use your elbows to gently push your knees outward, helping to open up your hips.

5. Lengthen your spine and keep your chest lifted, looking straight ahead or slightly upward.

6. Hold this pose for 30 seconds to 1 minute while taking deep breaths.

7. To release, place your hands on the ground in front of you, straighten your legs, and stand up.

40. Locust Pose:

Locust Pose is a great way to strengthen your back muscles. Here's how to perform it:

1. Lie flat on your stomach with your arms resting alongside your body, palms facing up.

2. Place your forehead on the mat, keeping your legs together.

3. Inhale as you lift your head, chest, arms, and legs off the mat simultaneously. Use your lower back muscles to lift your legs as high as you can.

4. Keep your gaze down to protect your neck and maintain a slight tuck of your chin.

5. Engage your buttocks and the muscles of your lower back to keep your legs lifted.

6. Hold this position for a few deep breaths, feeling the strength building in your back and legs.

7. Exhale as you slowly lower your body back down to the mat.

8. Repeat this pose a few times to build strength in your back muscles.

CONCLUSION

In the quiet space of our practice today, we've embarked on a journey of self-discovery, healing, and profound connection. Somatic yoga isn't just about the physical postures; it's a dance between body and soul, a gentle exploration of the wisdom within. As you move through each pose, you have taken steps towards greater awareness and harmony.

In the gentle sway of your breath, the softness of your movements, and the whispers of your body, you've unearthed the immense power of presence. Somatic yoga has invited you to listen deeply to your inner landscape, to honor your body's wisdom, and to embrace the beauty of your being.

Remember that this practice is a gift you can offer yourself every day, a sanctuary of self-love and self-acceptance. Let the lessons you've learned on your mat ripple into your life, nurturing a sense of peace, balance, and wholeness.

Dear Yogis,

I want to extend my heartfelt gratitude to each one of you for joining today's somatic yoga session. Your presence and dedication have illuminated our practice and created a beautiful, shared space of healing and growth.

Yoga is a journey, and it's the community that makes it even more enriching. Your commitment to self-care and self-discovery inspires me every day. I am honored to be a part of your wellness journey, and I look forward to sharing more moments of mindful movement and connection with you in the future.

As we continue on this path, may we always find solace and strength in the practice, and may it bring us closer to the radiant beings we truly are.

With deep appreciation and love,

DR PERSIS HILLARY...

BONUS: CONCLUSION

Day 1: Foundation Building

- Exercise: Begin with a 15-minute session of basic yoga stretches, including Child's Pose, Downward Dog, and Cat-Cow.

Day 2: Balance and Breath

- Exercise: Practice Tree Pose for balance and incorporate Ujjayi Pranayama (ocean breath) for breath control. Hold each pose for 30 seconds.

Day 3: Core Strength

- Exercise: Engage your core with Plank Pose, Boat Pose, and Leg Raises. Hold each for 30 seconds and repeat 2-3 times.

Day 4: Gentle Flow

- Exercise: Flow through a Sun Salutation sequence, focusing on smooth transitions and deep breaths. Repeat 5 rounds.

Day 5: Hip Opening

- Exercise: Perform Pigeon Pose, Butterfly Pose, and Happy Baby Pose to open up the hips. Hold each pose for 30 seconds.

Day 6: Twisting and Detoxifying

- Exercise: Practice seated and standing twists such as Seated Spinal Twist and Revolved Triangle Pose. Hold each for 30 seconds on each side.

Day 7: Rest and Restore

- Exercise: Take a day off for restorative yoga. Practice relaxation and meditation for 20 minutes.

Day 8: Strength and Balance

- Exercise: Incorporate Warrior I, II, and III poses into your practice. Hold each for 30 seconds and repeat 2-3 times.

Day 9: Backbends

- Exercise: Try Cobra Pose, Bridge Pose, and Camel Pose for back flexibility and strength. Hold each pose for 30 seconds.

Day 10: Deep Stretching

- Exercise: Focus on seated forward bends and stretches like Seated Forward Bend, Head-to-Knee Pose, and Butterfly Pose. Hold each for 30 seconds.

Day 11: Mindfulness Meditation

- Exercise: Dedicate today to mindfulness meditation. Start with 10 minutes and gradually increase your meditation time.

Day 12: Balance Challenge

- Exercise: Practice challenging balance poses like Half Moon Pose and Warrior III. Hold each for 30 seconds on each side.

Day 13: Inversions

- Exercise: Begin with Downward Dog and then attempt supported inversions like Legs Up the Wall or Shoulder Stand for 30 seconds.

Day 14: Rest and Recharge

- Exercise: Take a day off for rest and gentle stretching. Focus on self-care.

Day 15: Full Body Flow

- Exercise: Flow through a complete yoga sequence, combining strength, balance, and flexibility. Repeat 3-5 rounds.

Day 16: Hip and Quad Flexors

- Exercise: Practice poses like Low Lunge, Lizard Pose, and Quad Stretch to open up the hips and stretch the quads. Hold each for 30 seconds.

Day 17: Arm Strength

- Exercise: Work on arm strength with Chaturanga Dandasana, Crow Pose, or Dolphin Pose. Hold each for 30 seconds and repeat 2-3 times.

Day 18: Balance and Breath Control

- Exercise: Balance with poses like Eagle Pose and incorporate Bhramari Pranayama (humming bee breath) for breath control. Hold each pose for 30 seconds.

Day 19: Restorative Yoga

- Exercise: Focus on restorative poses like Savasana, Supported Fish Pose, and Supta Baddha Konasana for deep relaxation.

Day 20: Core and Twists

- Exercise: Strengthen your core with Boat Pose and add Seated or Standing Twists. Hold each for 30 seconds on each side.

Day 21: Meditation

- Exercise: Dedicate time to meditation. Explore different techniques and focus on mindfulness.

Day 22: Strength and Flexibility

- Exercise: Incorporate poses like Warrior I, II, III, and Triangle Pose for both strength and flexibility. Hold each for 30 seconds.

Day 23: Backbends and Heart Openers

- Exercise: Practice Heart Opening poses like Camel Pose, Bridge Pose, and Cobra Pose. Hold each for 30 seconds.

Day 24: Yin Yoga

- Exercise: Explore Yin Yoga poses, holding each for 3-5 minutes for deep stretching and relaxation.

Day 25: Mindful Movement

- Exercise: Flow through a mindful yoga sequence, focusing on fluidity, breath, and presence. Repeat 5 rounds.

Day 26: Balance Challenge

- Exercise: Challenge your balance with poses like Half Moon Pose, Warrior III, and Tree Pose. Hold each for 30 seconds on each side.

Day 27: Inversions

- Exercise: Attempt full inversions like Headstand or Handstand for 30 seconds with proper support and guidance.

Day 28: Rest and Reflection

- Exercise: Take a day off for rest and self-reflection. Journal about your yoga journey so far.

Day 29: Strength and Core

- Exercise: Strengthen your core with Plank Pose, Side Plank, and Boat Pose. Hold each for 30 seconds and repeat 2-3 times.

Day 30: Full Body Flow

- Exercise: Flow through a dynamic sequence that encompasses the entire body. Repeat 3-5 rounds.

Day 31: Hip Flexors and Quadriceps

- Exercise: Focus on poses like Low Lunge, Pigeon Pose, and Quad Stretch to release tension in the hip flexors and quads. Hold each for 30 seconds.

Day 32: Arm Balance

- Exercise: Challenge yourself with advanced arm balancing poses like Crow Pose or Firefly Pose for 30 seconds.

Day 33: Breath and Meditation

- Exercise: Dedicate today to deepening your breath control and meditation practice. Explore different pranayama techniques.

Day 34: Yin Yoga

- Exercise: Dive back into Yin Yoga, holding poses for 3-5 minutes for profound stretching and relaxation.

Day 35: Mindful Flow

- Exercise: Practice a slow and mindful flow, concentrating on your breath and awareness. Repeat 5 rounds.

Day 36: Balance and Inversions

- Exercise: Challenge your balance with poses like Half Moon Pose and Handstand. Hold each for 30 seconds on each side.

Day 37: Backbends and Heart Openers

- Exercise: Deepen your backbend practice with poses like Camel Pose, Wheel Pose, and Bow Pose. Hold each for 30 seconds.

Day 38: Full Body Yin

- Exercise: A gentle Yin Yoga session to release tension and prepare for the final days of the challenge.

Day 39: Celebration Flow

- Exercise: Flow through a joyful and celebratory sequence, acknowledging the progress you've made. Repeat 3-5 rounds.

Day 40: Gratitude and Reflection

- Exercise: On the final day, practice gratitude and reflection in Savasana

. Take time to appreciate your yoga journey and set intentions for the future.